The elderly rheumatic patient – diagnostic, prognostic and therapeutic aspects

D1827273

CIBA–GEIGY

Where research in antirheumatics
and services to the medical profession
go hand in hand

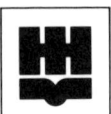

George E. Ehrlich and Guido Gallacchi

Editors

The elderly rheumatic patient – diagnostic, prognostic and therapeutic aspects

Report of a symposium held during the
XIth European Congress of Rheumatology,
Athens, 1987

Hans Huber Publishers
Toronto · Lewiston N.Y. · Bern · Stuttgart

Contents

Participants

Chairmen

GEORGE E. EHRLICH*, Medical Department, Ciba-Geigy Ltd,
Basle, Switzerland
* Now at: One Independence Place, Apt 1101, Sixth Street and Locust Walk,
Philadelphia, PA 19106.3731, USA

GUIDO GALLACCHI, Schmerzklinik Kirschgarten, Basle, Switzerland

Speakers

JAN DEQUEKER, Afd Reumatologie, Universitaire Zuikenhuizen Leuven
uz Pellenberg, Belgium

GEORGE NUKI, Rheumatic Diseases Unit, University of Edinburgh,
Northern General Hospital, Edinburgh, UK

RAFFAELE NUMO, Centro di Medicina Sociale di Reumatologia,
Bari, Italy

JACQUES PEYRON, Centre de Rhumatologie, Hôpital de la Pitié,
Paris, France

Preface

Arthritis and other rheumatic disorders are common among the elderly. Yet the passage of years alone is not responsible for all the abnormalities of the musculoskeletal system manifested with increasing age. This symposium therefore considers the many other factors concerned in their causation, as well as their diagnosis, prognosis and therapy.

The recent growth of interest in geriatric medicine reflects more than increasing longevity and an ageing population structure. It also recognises that the years produce changes in every physiological function, although not at the same rate, and certainly not equally in all individuals. Some would argue that growing older is normal, ageing abnormal. Certainly, distinctions must be drawn which serve to identify pathological changes in good time. The implications are not that we can perpetuate youth but that some of the decline should be preventable.

The decline in muscles and joints starts quite early in life, from the end of the second decade, usually beginning to become clinically apparent in the fourth decade. Of all the physiological systems, the musculoskeletal is the earliest to evince such changes. In most forms of athletics, the participant is considered old before the 40th birthday. Early traumata, imbalances of alignment or structure, inflammatory diseases such as rheumatoid arthritis, and conditions of later years such as Paget's disease, hyperthyroidism, parathyroidism, osteoporosis, and other metabolic disorders all contribute to the number of elderly sufferers from diverse musculoskeletal problems.

The resulting accumulation of musculoskeletal disability in the elderly accounts for a major share of social isolation, pain, and quiet desperation. But we have begun to realise in recent years that the disabling effects of such conditions are not all inevitable. Geriatrics and gerontology now recognise that old people are not just young people wearing out as the years pass. Specific physical, physiological, and psychological changes take place with ageing and need to be taken into account for the attempted remedy to be optimal.

Many questions therefore arise in considering the elderly rheumatic patient. What can be accepted as 'normal' loss of function? Can any markers be identified which would show us when age-related changes are becoming pathological? Which early symptoms are functionally relevant and require specific investigation and treatment? Is it possible to identify older patients in whom the prognosis is poor (e.g. measures of decrepitude)? Should specific therapy be started in such patients, when symptomatic relief may do more to increase their quality of life, in keeping with their reduced life-expectancy? How does the complex spectrum of ageing processes influence the causation and development of joint pathology and the treatment of arthritis and other rheumatological conditions in the elderly?

These are among the important questions discussed at this symposium – and now brought to a wider medical audience – by specialists distinguished for their work on different aspects of rheumatic disease in the elderly.

G. E. Ehrlich
G. Gallacchi

The ageing joint – normal and abnormal changes

JACQUES G. PEYRON
Centre de Rhumatologie, Hôpital de la Pitié, Paris, France

Summary

The ageing joint usually maintains its capacity for efficient mobility under load. However, with the passage of time, an increasing number of joints in an increasing number of subjects undergo osteoarthritic changes, which proceed more rapidly after the age of 50. The possible mechanisms that underlie this proneness to OA are being studied at the site of its earliest known lesions in the articular cartilage. Many of these changes differ from those that occur in ageing cartilage.

In spite of some interesting preliminary observations, changes in the articular cartilage of elderly subjects have not yet shed much light on proneness to develop OA. This may be partly because ageing is instrumental in the inception of OA only when associated with other factors: excessive or improper mechanical stress, heredity, and perhaps inflammation. But since ageing is the most consistent and widespread risk factor for OA, its study is of the utmost practical importance.

Introduction

The normal ageing joint usually maintains its capacity for movement under weight-bearing conditions with extremely low friction, in spite of a certain degree of limitation of mobility due to increased stiffness of periarticular structures (muscles, ligaments, capsules). Functional surface smoothness and biomechanical properties of the articular cartilage generally remain good.

However, an increasing number of joints in an increasing number of subjects undergo osteoarthritic changes as time goes by. This age-related proneness to osteoarthritis is clearly borne out by clinical observation (PEYRON, 1984). Radiological evidence of osteoarthritis in at least one joint is present in 2% of women below 45 years, 30% between 45 and 65, and 68% after 65. In men, the corresponding figures are 3%, 24.5% and 58%, respectively.

Moreover, this increase is uneven. Slow and arithmetical until 50–55 years, it becomes rapid and geometrical thereafter (Fig. 1), suggesting that the effects of several factors could be combined during the later period. Indeed, extrinsic causes of osteoarthritis, mostly mechanical, which predominate in early cases, become less prevalent with the onset of osteoarthritis, which is usually 'primary' in appearance among elderly people.

11

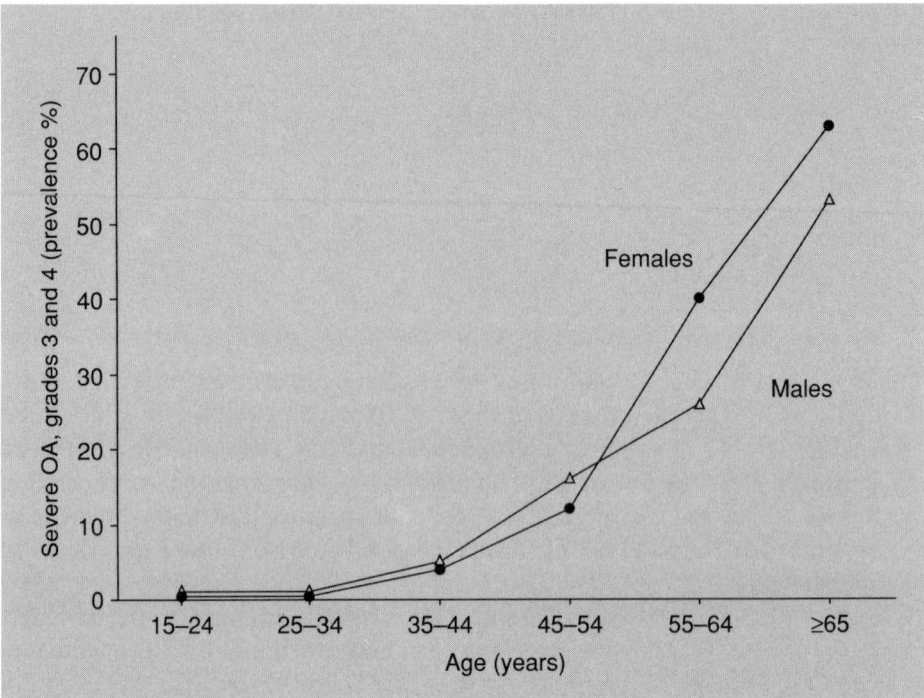

Fig. 1. Correlation of OA with age in at least one joint among males and females from two English population samples. (Data from Lawrence, J.S., *Rheumatism in Populations,* Heinemann Medical Books, 1977. Reprinted from Peyron, 1984, with permission of the publisher.)

There is thus a sound case for studying the mechanisms that underlie this propensity of ageing joints to develop osteoarthritis. Since articular cartilage is the earliest and main target of the osteoarthritic lesions, this paper will focus on the changes – anatomical, biophysical, biochemical and enzymatic – that are known to occur in ageing cartilage.

Anatomical changes

Anatomical changes in the ageing hip have been described as an increase in congruence between the femoral head and the acetabulum (BULLOUGH et al, 1973); thus, the usual mechanism of adaptation to increased load, which consists in extending the area of contact between the two surfaces, is impaired. Maintenance of the physiological degree of incongruence through-out a person's life is an active process, pressure dependent, entailing a slow and permanent remodelling of the bone-cartilage junction (GOODFELLOW and MITSOU, 1977). This mechanism could be impaired in certain ageing subjects. However, moulding of the joint cavity of human hips under pres-

12

sure has shown that joint conformation is in fact very variable and does not display a systematic decrease in older specimens (AFOKE et al, 1983).

Thickening of extensor tendons of the finger has been mentioned as a factor which contributes to interphalangeal osteoarthritis in elderly people (SMYTHE, 1985).

Another age-linked systemic factor that could jeopardise joint function is impairment of the fine control of joint position and movement, due to a decrease of proprioceptive sensitivity. This has been documented in elderly subjects and is even more diminished in patients with osteoarthritis of the knee (SKINNER et al, 1984).

The thickness of articular cartilage does not change with age. The cell density decreases in the superficial upper middle layers in the femoral head (VIGNON et al, 1976) and in the femoral condyle (QUINTERO et al, 1984). This might impair the capacity of articular cartilage to respond to a new situation by manufacturing enough new components.

Ageing cartilage is slightly discoloured, becoming faintly yellowish instead of white. This is more marked in costal cartilage and is due to a pigment of unknown origin (VAN DER KORST et al, 1968).

On surface examination, non-osteoarthritic joints display areas of roughness and shallow erosions. These changes increase in frequency over the years but not much in extent or depth, and are therefore described as 'non-progressive lesions' (BYERS et al, 1970). They are mainly seen in the non-weight-bearing, usually peripheral, zones of articular cartilage. In the femoral head they can be distinguished with relative ease from early osteoarthritic lesions, though the difference is less clear in the knee.

The matrix of ageing cartilage displays some slight changes, such as irregularities or a reduplication of the 'tide-mark' in places. Possibly more significant is the existence of some surface irregularities, better seen on scanning electron microscopy, which reveals unmasking of surface fibrillar bundles (LONGMORE and GARDNER, 1975). These surface changes might alter the efficiency of the lubricating mechanism in the ageing joint (UNSWORTH, 1984).

Biophysical changes

Specimens of articular cartilage from elderly people have been shown to undergo some biophysical changes. A decrease of tensile strength (i.e. resistance to fracture oriented along the superficial fibres) has been repeatedly documented (KEMPSON, 1975; ROBERTS et al, 1986). This feature is due directly to deterioration in the integrity of the collagen network, with diminished resistance to stress.

The existence of age-related changes in tensile stiffness (the amount of strain for a given stress) and in compressive stiffness – features more related to the interfibrillar components of the matrix – is more controversial.

Subchondral bone density has been found to be decreased in the lower pole of femoral heads of elderly subjects but not in the upper, weight-bearing region (ROBERTS et al, 1986).

Biochemical changes

Any change in the properties of ageing articular cartilage must depend on some alteration to its biochemical composition. The changes that have been documented in this field are summarised in Tables I and II, and compared to those that have been found in osteoarthritic cartilage.

How these changes increase proneness to osteoarthritis is unclear. In fact, several changes, particularly the decrease in water content, are the opposite of those found in the early stages of osteoarthritic degradation. However, several recent studies have disclosed some stimulating observations.

On one hand, proteoglycans in ageing cartilage have been shown to be more poorly aggregated (ROUGHLEY et al, 1984), with the most highly buoyant density aggregates being lost (MANICOURT et al, 1986). This could be related, at least in part, to a loss of functional efficiency of the link proteins (MORT et al, 1983). Proteoglycans poorly aggregated could be more easily driven out of the matrix by mechanical forces.

Table I. Features of the ageing joint – comparison with osteoarthritis. Changes in cartilage collagens and glycosaminoglycans.

	Ageing	Osteoarthritis
Collagen II (FUJII, 1975)		
– content	Unchanged	Unchanged
– solubility	Decreased	Increased
Collagen IX (HERBAGE, 1986)		
– content	Decreased	
Water content (VENN, 1978)	Decreased	Increased
Chondroitin sulphate (HJERTQUIST and LEMPERG, 1972)		
– content	Unchanged	Decreased
– chain length	Decreased	Increased, then decreased
– C45/C65	Decreased	Increased
Keratan sulphate (HJERTQUIST and LEMPERG, 1972)		
– content	Increased	Decreased
Hyaluronic acid (GARDNER et al, 1980)		
– content	Increased	Decreased

Table II. Features of the ageing joint – comparison with osteoarthritis. Changes in proteoglycans (PG).

	Ageing	Osteoarthritis
PG content (BAYLISS and ALI, 1978)	Unchanged	Decreased
PG extractability (BAYLISS and ALI, 1978)	Decreased	Increased
Monomer size (BAYLISS and ALI, 1978)	Decreased	Decreased
Aggregation (ROUGHLEY et al, 1984)	Decreased	Decreased
Hyaluronic acid binding region (HABR) (ROUGHLEY et al, 1985)		
– rate of maturation	Decreased	Increased
– free HABR	Increased	
Small non-aggregated PG (PEYRON et al, 1978)	Decreased	Decreased
Link proteins (MORT et al, 1983)	Fragmented	

On the other hand, some ancillary factors of the fibrillar network cohesiveness, such as collagen IX, may be deficient in old cartilage (HERBAGE, 1986). This could confer a certain degree of fragility to the collagen architecture, not fully explained otherwise. Collagen II, the main constituent, remains quantitatively normal and even less soluble (i.e. more cross-linked) in old specimens.

Finally, the loss of some species of small, non-aggregated proteoglycans (STANESCU, 1987) might be deleterious in some way to the interaction between matrix and fibrils, a feature not yet understood.

All these defects could render ageing cartilage more susceptible to mechanical damage under a given mechanical stress. It is still uncertain whether they imply faulty collagen synthesis, or some degradative activity, or both.

The changes observed in the main type of glycosaminoglycans within the proteoglycans could reflect the progressive replacement of one population of proteoglycan by another in early adulthood (GLANT et al, 1986).

Enzyme changes

Degradating enzymes, acidic proteases, neutral proteoglycanases and collagenase activity have not been found to be increased in cartilage from old subjects (MARTEL-PELLETIER and PELLETIER, 1987). Regarding synthesis, one recent study showed that articular cartilages from old cows produced an equal amount of proteoglycans but significantly less collagen and glycopro-

15

teins when compared with those of young calves (MITROVIC et al, 1986). In osteoarthritic cartilage all enzymic activities, synthetic and degradative, are increased.

Conclusions

Thus, despite a few stimulating preliminary indications, we still understand little of why the joint tissues of elderly subjects are increasingly liable to develop osteoarthritis. Present evidence suggests that the osteoarthritic process (or processes) is not an exaggeration or an indirect effect of ageing, but probably implies some superimposed mechanism(s). However, a certain decrease in the cohesiveness of the matrix could constitute an age-linked risk factor.

Ageing is instrumental in the inception of OA only when associated with other aetiological factors: mechanical insults, hormonal and body-building status, probably heredity, perhaps associated with inflammation and/or some metabolic disturbance. However, ageing itself is the most prominent risk factor in joint changes, as both individuals and populations get older. Study of its mechanisms of action therefore remains of the utmost practical importance.

References

AFOKE, N.Y.P., BYERS, P.D. and HUTTON, W.C. (1983) The incongruous hip joint: a loading study. *Ann. Rheum. Dis. 43*, 295–301.

BAYLISS, M.T. and ALI, S. (1978) Age-related changes in the composition and structure of human articular cartilage proteoglycans. *Biochem. J. 176*, 683–693.

BULLOUGH, P., GOODFELLOW, J. and O'CONNOR, J. (1973) The relationship between degenerative changes and load bearing in the human hip. *J. Bone Joint Surg. 55B*, 746–758.

BYERS, P., CONTEPOMI, C.A. and FARKAS, T.A. (1970) Post-mortem study of the hip joint. *Ann. Rheum. Dis. 29*, 15–31.

FUJII, K. (1975) Ageing of the collagen in human joint components. Changes in the reducible cross-links and solubilities. *J. Jpn. Orthop. Assoc. 49*, 145–155.

GARDNER, D.L., ELLIOT, R.J., ARMSTRONG, C.G. et al (1980) The relationship between age, thickness, surface structure, compliance and composition of human head articular cartilage. In: *The Aetiopathogenesis of Osteoarthritis*, pp. 65–83 (Ed. G. Nuki). Pitman Medical, Tunbridge Wells.

GLANT, T.T., MIKECZ, K., ROUGHLEY, P.J. et al (1986) Age-related changes in protein-related epitopes of human articular cartilage proteoglycans. *Biochem. J. 236*, 71–75.

GOODFELLOW, J. and MITSOU, A. (1977) Joint surface incongruity and its maintenance. An experimental study. *J. Bone Joint Surg. 59A*, 446–451.

HERBAGE, D. (1986) Role of minor collagens in cartilage matrix organization (discussion). In: *Degenerative Joint Disease*, p. 14. Report of an International Symposium held 21–23 October 1986. The Kennedy Institute of Rheumatology, London.

HJERTQUIST, S.O. and LEMPERG, R. (1972) Identification and concentration of the glycosaminoglycans of human articular cartilage in relation to age and osteoarthritis. *Calcif. Tissue Res. 10*, 223–237.

KEMPSON, G. E. (1975) Mechanical properties of articular cartilage and their relation to matrix degradation and age. *Ann. Rheum. Dis. 34* (Suppl. 2), 111–113.

LONGMORE, R. B. and GARDNER, D. L. (1975) Development with age of human articular cartilage surface structure. A survey by interference microscopy of the lateral femoral condyle. *Ann. Rheum. Dis. 34,* 26–37.

MANICOURT, D. H., PITA, J. C., PEZON, C. F. et al (1986) Characterization of the proteoglycans recovered under non-dissociative conditions from normal articular cartilage of rabbits and dogs. *J. Biol. Chem. 261,* 5426–5433.

MARTEL-PELLETIER, J. and PELLETIER, J.-P. (1987) Neutral metalloproteases and age-related changes in human articular cartilage. *Ann. Rheum. Dis. 46,* 363–369.

MITROVIC, D., SWANN, D. A., FRONT, P. et al (1986) Protein-glycoprotein-collagen but not proteoglycan synthesis is deficient in aged, bovine articular cartilage. Possible implications in osteoarthritis (abstract). *XV Symp. Europ. Soc. Osteoarthrology,* Kuopio. Held 25–27 June 1986, Abstr. A5.

MORT, J. S., POOLE, A. R. and ROUGHLEY, P. J. (1983) Age-related changes in the structure of proteoglycan link proteins present in normal human articular cartilage. *Biochem. J. 214,* 269–272.

PEYRON, J. G. (1984) The epidemiology of osteoarthritis. In: *Osteoarthritis: Diagnosis and Management,* pp. 9–27 (Eds. R. W. Moskowitz et al). Saunders, Philadelphia.

PEYRON, J. G., STANESCU, R., STANESCU, V. et al (1978) Distribution électrophorétique particulière des populations de protéoglycanes dans les zones de régénération du cartilage arthrosique et étude de leur collagène. *Rev. Rhum. Mal. Osteoart. 45,* 569–575.

QUINTERO, M., MITROVIC, D. R., STANKOVIC, A. et al (1984) Aspects cellulaires du vieillissement du cartilage articulaire. I. Cartilage condylien à surface normale, prélevé dans des genoux normaux. *Rev. Rhumat. 51,* 375–379.

ROBERTS, S., WEIGHTMAN, B., URBAN, J. et al (1986) Mechanical and biochemical properties of human articular cartilage in osteoarthritic femoral heads and in autopsy specimens. *J. Bone Joint Surg. 68B,* 278–288.

ROUGHLEY, P. J., WHITE, R. J. and POOLE, A. R. (1985) Identification of a hyaluronic acid binding protein that interferes with the preparation of high buoyant density proteoglycan aggregates from adult human articular cartilage. *Biochem. J. 231,* 129–138.

ROUGHLEY, P. J., WHITE, R. J., POOLE, A. R. et al (1984) The inability to prepare high buoyant density proteoglycan aggregates from extracts of normal adult human articular cartilage. *Biochem. J. 221,* 637–644.

SKINNER, H. B., BARRACK, R. L., COOK, S. D. et al (1984) Joint position sense in total knee arthroplasty. *J. Orthop. Res. 1,* 276–283.

SMYTHE, H. A. (1985) The mechanical pathogenesis of generalized osteoarthritis. In: *Osteoarthritis, Current Clinical and Fundamental Problems,* p. 6671 (Ed. J. G. Peyron). Ciba-Geigy, Paris.

STANESCU, Y. (1987) Changes in the chemistry of proteoglycans with ageing. In: *Eurorhumatology,* pp. 107–109 (Eds. A. Andrianakos et al). XIth Europ. Congress Rheumatol., Athens.

UNSWORTH, A. (1984) Some biochemical factors in osteoarthrosis. In: *Joint Failure.* First Scientif. Meet. Br. Soc. Rheumatol., 4–6 April, 1984.

VAN DER KORST, J. K., SOKOLOFF, L. and MILLER E. J. (1968) Senescent pigmentation of cartilage and degenerative joint disease. *Arch. Pathol. 86,* 40–47.

VENN, M. F. (1978) Variation of chemical composition with age in human femoral head cartilage. *Ann. Rheum. Dis. 37,* 168–174.

VIGNON, E., ARLOT, M. and VIGNON, G. (1976) Etude de la densité cellulaire du cartilage de la tête fémorale en fonction de l'âge. *Rev. Rhumatol. 43,* 403–405.

17

Triggering factors for pathological joint changes

JAN DEQUEKER

Department of Rheumatology, University of Leuven, Pellenberg, Belgium

Summary

Whatever the prime causes of osteoarthritis, rheumatoid disease and other articular disorders eventually prove to be, the onset and expression of joint changes are governed by many factors. These can be categorised under main headings as age-related, genetic, hormonal, environmental, and associated with intercurrent disease. Recognition of their effects should facilitate suitable preventive and/or therapeutic measures – with prospects of deferring joint damage and minimising its effects. Among patterns of joint disease associated with ageing, osteoarthritis and osteoporosis – both common in the elderly – seldom if ever coexist in the same patient.

A broad range of life events and other factors influence the expression of certain joint disorders and their response to treatment, as outlined below.

Host susceptibility

Individual predisposition, whether inherited or acquired, often appears to play a part in determining the type of disorder a patient develops and/or the clinical form it takes. Chondrocalcinosis is typical of a disease in which various different triggering factors lead to different kinds of syndrome: pseudogout, pseudo-rheumatoid arthritis, pseudo-osteoarthrosis, pseudo-osteoarthrosis with acute attacks, asymptomatic calcium pyrophosphate deposition and pseudo-neuroarthropathy.

This complex picture of multiple causes and varied effects gives rise to fundamental questions: Why are the underlying changes expressed in different ways? What does the background predisposition to chondrocalcinosis consist of, and how is it triggered into clinical disease? There is certainly a genetic element. Polyarticular chondrocalcinosis is known to occur in some families. At the same time, chondrocalcinosis is much more frequent in the ageing than in the younger population. Hormones may be involved – chondrocalcinosis is certainly associated with hyperparathyroidism, with acromegaly and probably also with diabetes. The different clinical patterns of chondrocalcinosis may also be due to the effects of intercurrent disease on osteoarthritis and other joint disorders or to changes in sensory neurological structure.

Biomechanics and joint congruity

Mechanical factors that impose stresses on a joint or impair its congruity play a role in triggering the development of articular disease – and in its expression. One patient with a paralysed arm due to a traumatic nerve section developed very marked radiological signs of rheumatoid arthritis in the opposite, non-paralysed limb, which was doubtless exposed to extra work. The paralysed limb showed no joint deterioration, although there was a subcutaneous nodule on that elbow. Another patient came to our clinic with very severe rheumatoid arthritis, never previously seen by a doctor. His X-rays showed markedly cystic lesions, characteristic of rheumatoid disease but also reflecting exposure to mechanical factors, as seen in the so-called robust-type rheumatoid arthritis.

Factors such as Paget's disease which change the congruity of the hip joint will lead to osteoarthritis. Aseptic necrosis, unless it is seen early and steps are taken to protect against cartilage destruction, will lead to early osteoarthritis of the hip. These examples may serve to make the general points that mechanical stresses on a joint both increase the risk of developing osteo-arthritis and influence the way in which any articular disease is manifested.

Ageing, immunology, and sex differences

These factors are often considered separately, but some immunological changes are known to be age-related, notably a decline in thymic function, reduced response to primary antigen challenge, and lowering of both antibody production and delayed hypersensitivity. Responses to secondary (or delayed) hypersensitivity are also reduced with age; at the same time, homoeostatic control tends to decline, with rising autoantibody levels and increased frequency of benign monoclonal gamma-globulinopathies.

Sex appears to play a role in those oligoarthritic conditions, the seronegative osteoarthropathies, which occur mainly in the younger age group, of either sex (Fig. 1), with a tendency for the spine to be involved more in men and the peripheral joints in women (Table I) (DEQUEKER et al, 1978a). The rheumatic conditions associated with autoimmunity are, by contrast, more prevalent in the elderly. Ageing on its own certainly has a profound effect on the incidence of osteoporosis, especially in postmenopausal females; at the same time there is an age-related increase in the prevalence of osteoarthrosis, more so in females than in males (Fig. 1). But these two conditions seldom occur together in elderly women.

It has long been known that elderly patients who fracture the neck of the femur have well-preserved femoral heads and articular cartilage, while those who have osteoarthritis of the hip joint do not break the femoral neck. Similarly in the spine, patients with disc lesions and osteophyte formation have well-preserved vertebrae and bone structure, whereas the osteoporotic patients liable to fractures and vertebral collapse have well-preserved discs

Table I. The chronic inflammatory rheumatic diseases: HLA-B27 and sex ratio.

Rheumatoid condition	HLA-B27 (%)	Male:female ratio
Rheumatoid arthritis		
☐ Seropositive	6	1 : 3.5
☐ Seronegative	40	1 : 2.6
Ankylosing spondylitis		
☐ Bamboo spine	39	1 : 0.2
☐ Syndesmophytes + peripheral arthritis	89	1 : 1.6
☐ Syndesmophytes minus peripheral arthritis	91	1 : 0.8
Juvenile chronic arthritis	58	1 : 0.9
Reiter	56	1 : 0.4
Inflammatory bowel disease + arthritis	40	1 : 0.4
Psoriatic arthritis	17	1 : 1.3
Yersinia arthritis	53	1 : 0.9

with very little or no osteophyte formation. *So among the elderly there are two populations: those with a rather atrophic type of bone which fractures easily, and those with a more hypertrophic type of bone who develop cartilage disease and osteoarthritis* (DEQUEKER, 1985).

Menopausal and other endocrine influences

Around the menopause several rheumatic conditions commonly come to expression: nodular generalised osteoarthrosis, characterised by Heberden's nodes, seropositive rheumatoid arthritis, and (only after the menopause) gout (Fig. 1). What effect do estrogens have on osteoarthrosis? We looked at a population of menopausal women who had taken estrogen substitution therapy for more than five years and graded the changes at the hand joints before and after treatment. We did not find any difference compared to the rest of the population (Fig. 2). So estrogen alone does not protect against the development of osteoarthrosis, at least in the small hand joints (DEQUEKER et al, 1978b).

Estrogens do appear to have a profound effect on rheumatoid arthritis; no new cases occur during pregnancy, and oral contraceptives have also been shown to have some protective effect against its development (VANDEN-BROUCKE et al, 1982). Also, estrogens definitely play an important part in normal bone and calcium metabolism.

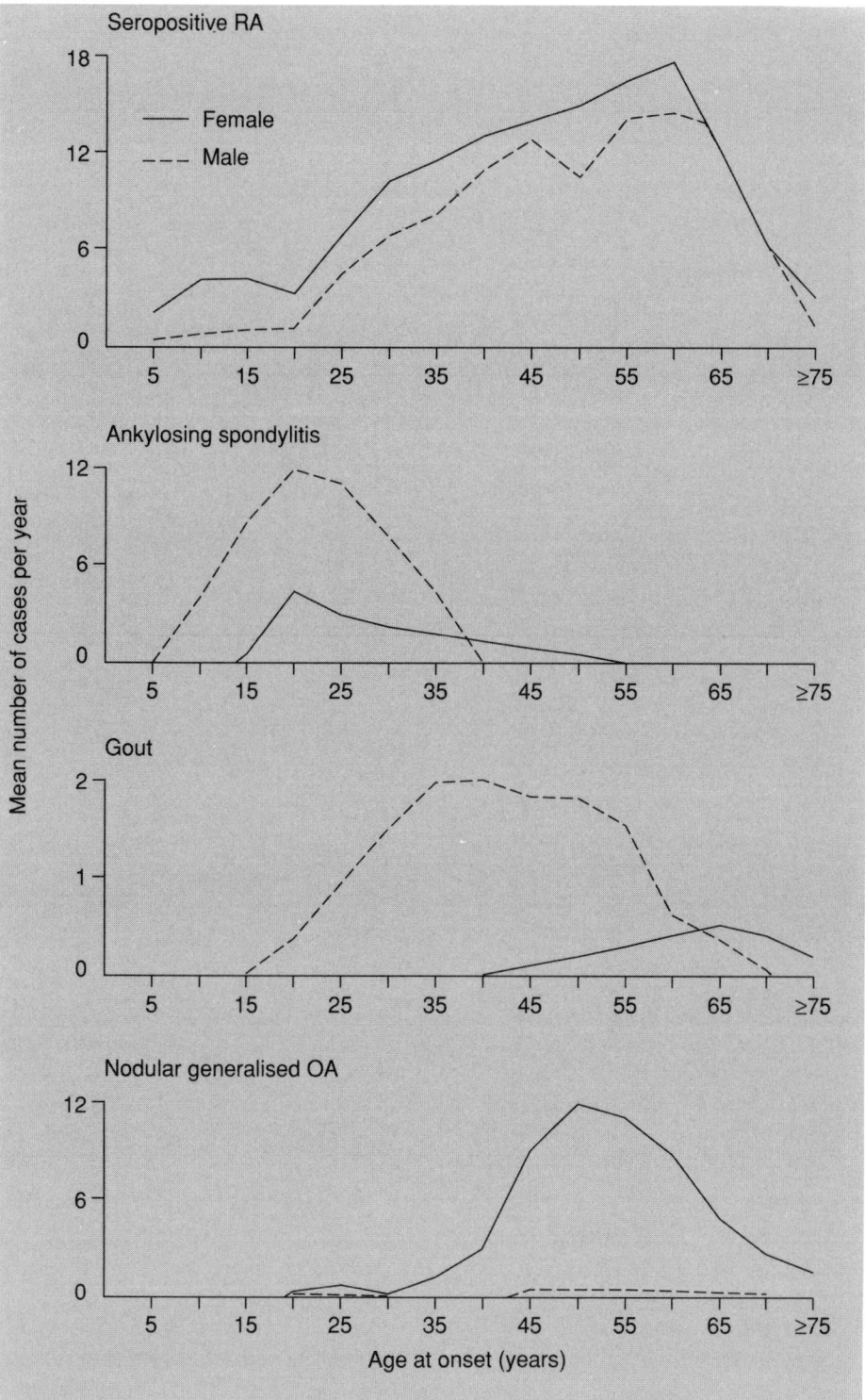

Fig. 1. Age and sex distribution of four major types of rheumatic disease.

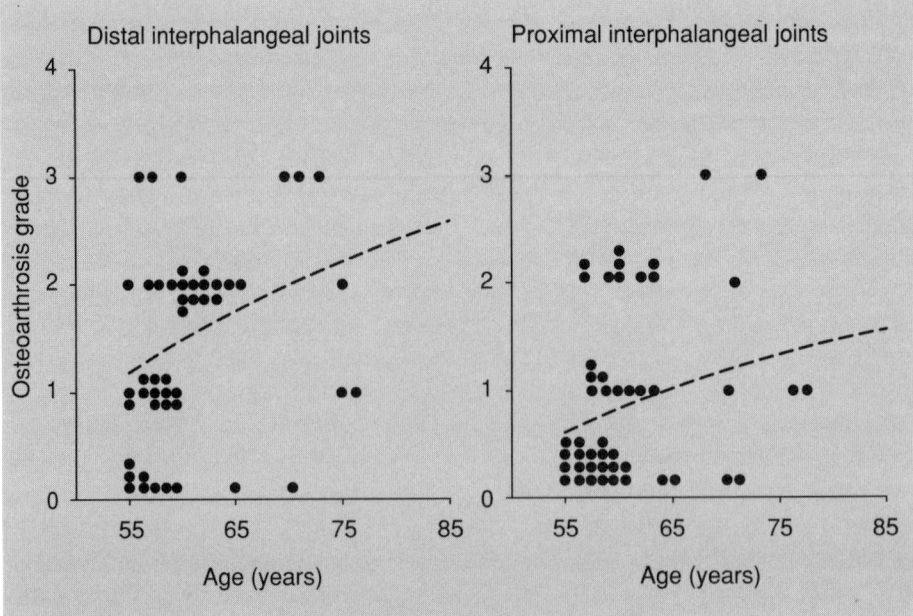

Estrogen treatment more than 5 years

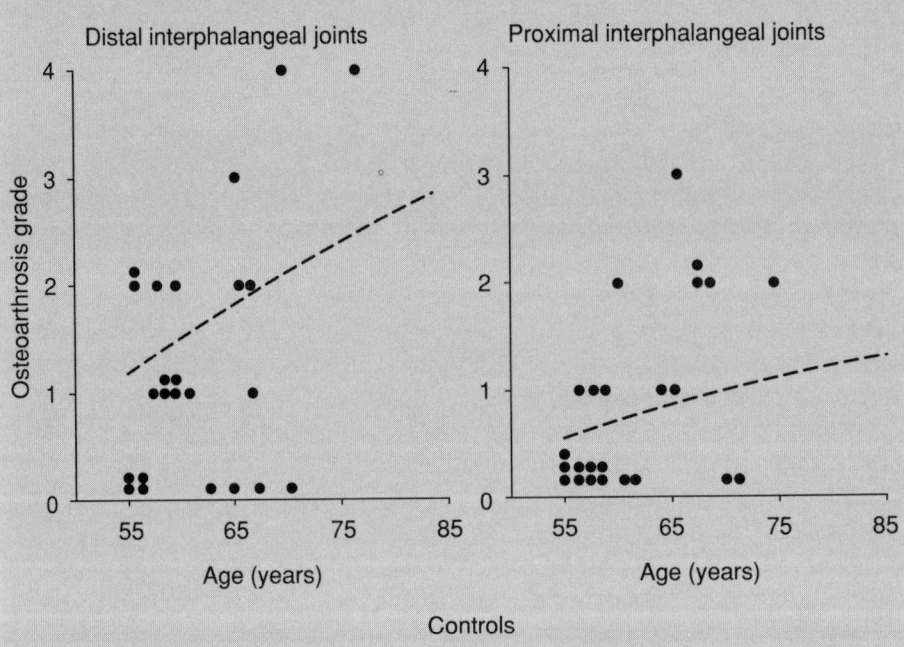

Fig. 2. Osteoarthrosis of distal and proximal interphalangeal joints in postmenopausal women, showing that estrogen substitution therapy for over five years has no effect on severity, compared with controls.

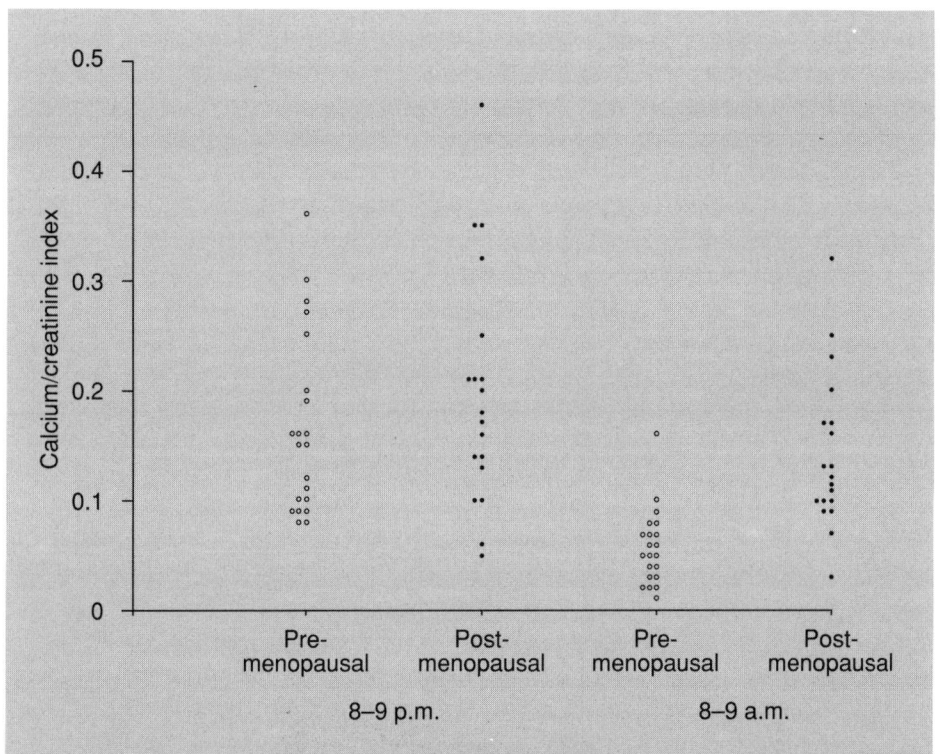

Fig. 3. Sensitivity of bone to parathyroid hormone changes after the menopause, as demonstrated by determining the calcium:creatinine ratio in fasting urine *(right)*, but not in evening specimens *(left)*.

Immediately after the menopause, natural or surgical, the sensitivity of bone to the action of parathyroid hormone is changed. This can be detected only by determining the calcium:creatinine ratio in the fasting urine; evening or 24-hour urine does not give such a clear picture (Fig. 3). The bone in our population study was measured at the metacarpals, the distal radius, and the lumbar spine, where trabecular bone predominates (Fig. 4). We found that the amount of bone in the spine was maximal at the age of 25, while cortical bone, measured in the radius, is maximal at the age of 40. Loss of spinal bone is very rapid after the menopause, but loss of cortical bone proceeds gradually with ageing (Fig. 5) (Geusens et al, 1986).

Not every woman over 50 will develop symptomatic osteoporosis. Even by the age of 80, only 25% of women will have sustained a fracture, usually of the spine, femur or wrist (Fig. 5). So who are the patients at risk? When do we need to identify them? At the age of 45–50, around the onset of the menopause, to prevent excessive bone loss, especially from the vertebral column.

One of the risk factors we studied was the anthropometrical constitution of postmenopausal patients, comparing osteoporotic cases to those with gener-

23

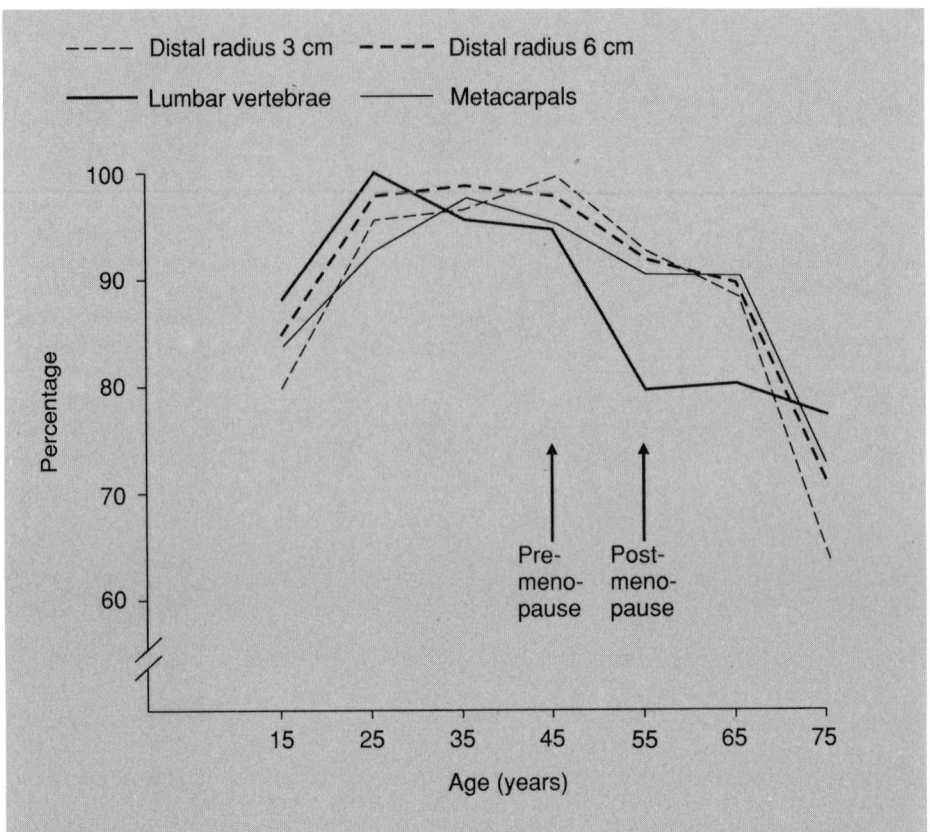

Fig. 4. The decline in peak bone mass from peak levels in the premenopausal years accelerates after the menopause. Note differences between metacarpal, radial and vertebral bone.

alised osteoarthrosis, who – as noted above – do not frequently develop vertebral or femoral neck fractures. The osteoarthrotic patients were found to have greater skinfold thickness than osteoporotic subjects of the same age, with more subcutaneous fat and significantly greater bodyweight, muscle power and muscle mass (DEQUEKER et al, 1983). Skinfold thickness is important after the menopause because it reflects the quantity of subcutaneous fat, where androstenedione from the ovaries and suprarenals is aromatised to estrone – which appears to be what protects osteoarthrotic women from part of the rapid calcium loss after the menopause.

Thus some excess of bodyweight after the menopause protects against osteoporosis, but also imposes stresses on weight-bearing joints including the lumbar spine, giving rise to back and neck pain. In fat women this back pain is not due to osteoporosis but to apophysial osteoarthritis and disc lesions.

Among other endocrine influences, growth hormone affects the expression of joint disease in acromegaly. Excessive growth hormone stimulates cartilage

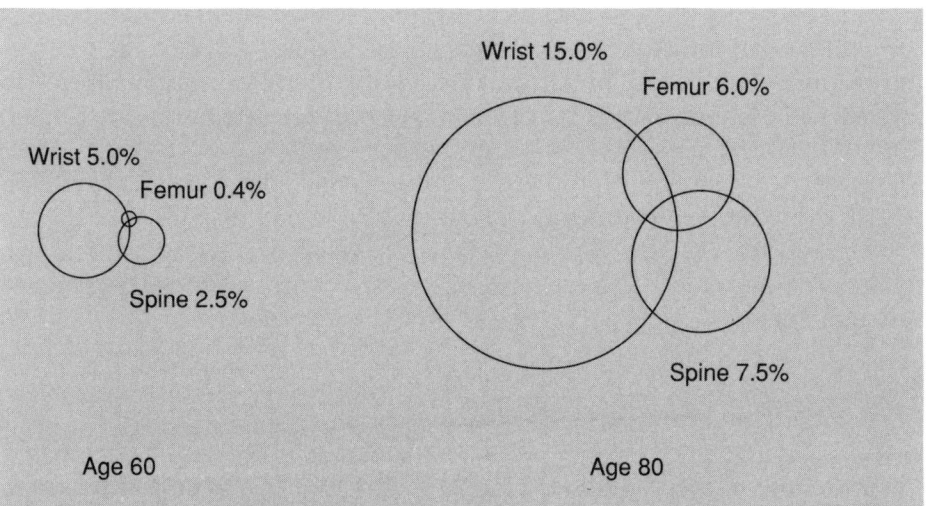

Fig. 5. Fractures of wrist, femur and spine in the postmenopausal population become markedly more frequent between the ages of 60 and 80 years.

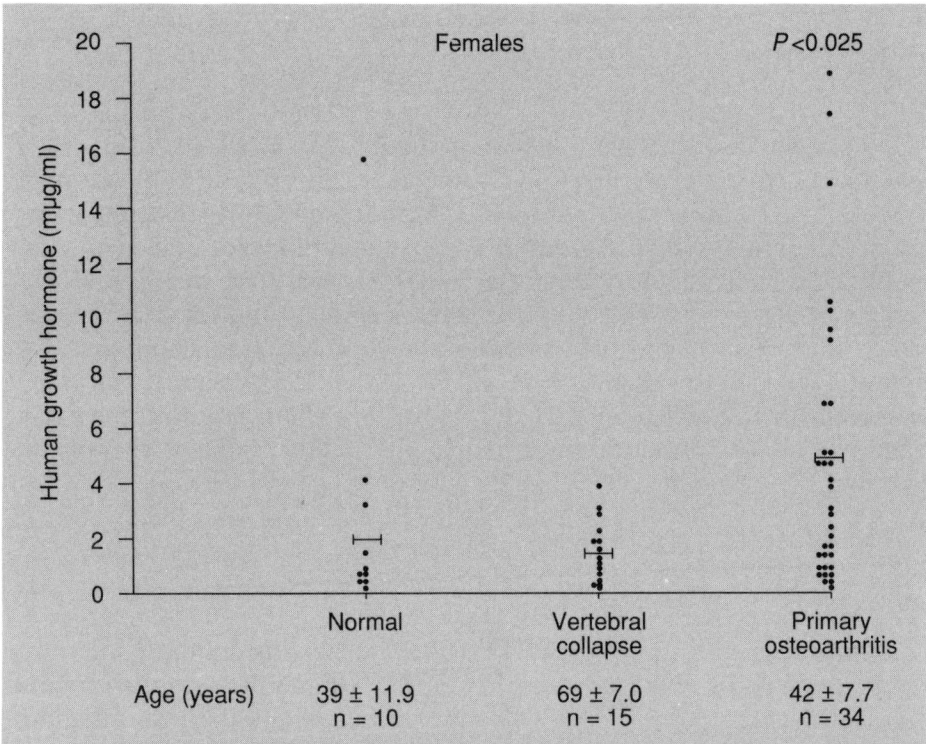

Fig. 6. Growth hormone levels in postmenopausal women, showing elevation in many cases of osteoarthritis, but no difference between normal subjects and those with vertebral collapse due to osteoporosis.

growth, producing the typical clinical and radiological picture of acromegalic hands and other joints. After some years these patients will develop osteoarthrosis of the hands, hip joints and knees. Growth hormone also appears to influence the changes seen in primary generalised osteoarthrosis (Fig. 6) (DEQUEKER et al, 1982).

The incidence of systemic lupus erythematosus (SLE) decreases in postmenopausal, compared with younger, women. Indeed late-onset SLE after the age of 50 is seen more in men than in women. Testosterone has also been shown, in New Zealand mice, to have a protective effect against the expression of systemic lupus.

Environment and lifestyle

The incidence of rheumatoid arthritis is higher in urban than in rural areas, and the further south we go, the less severely is it expressed. Rheumatoid arthritis is also reported to be less severe and its incidence lower in areas where malaria is prevalent. Thus, triggering of the immune system by infections or other factors might protect against the development of and/or modify the expression of such conditions.

Diet

Many patients ask what they should or should not eat vis-à-vis their rheumatoid arthritis, and we now have some answers. Dietetic antigens might provoke hypersensitivity responses (i.e. 'food allergies'), which could in turn lead to rheumatic symptoms. Second, nutritional modifications might alter immune and inflammatory responses and thus modify the manifestation of rheumatic disease. Patients taking fish-oil fatty acid supplementation experience alleviation of morning stiffness and joint swelling, compared with those taking placebo (KREMER et al, 1987). This is because unsaturated fish-oil fatty acids are competitive inhibitors for the formation of the prostaglandins and leukotrienes concerned in the pathogenesis of rheumatoid arthritis.

Drug therapy

Can drugs trigger off joint disease or aggravate existing damage? There are several main types of drug to consider: the disease-modifying antirheumatic drugs (gold, chloroquine, D-penicillamine), the non-steroidal anti-inflammatory drugs, and the pure analgesics.

Drugs such as procainamide and D-penicillamine have long been known to induce systemic lupus-like syndromes in some patients. For this there is a recognised genetic predisposition (HLA DR4) and also a slow acetylator phenotype which might act as an ancillary trigger factor (BATCHELOR et al, 1980). The role of HLA DR3 in adverse drug reactions to gold and penicillamine among rheumatoid arthritis patients – especially the occurrence of proteinurea – has given rise to much controversy and the association may not be as strong as suggested a few years ago (WOOLEY et al, 1980). Certainly, many HLA DR3 negative subjects do develop proteinurea (DEQUEKER et al, 1984). Another trigger factor, not related to the HLA DR status, is relative impairment of sulphoxidation.

Much has been written about the possible negative effects of non-steroidal anti-inflammatory drugs (NSAIDs) on cartilage and on proteoglycan synthesis and their positive action in inhibiting proteolytic enzymes. These two actions probably tend to cancel each other out. NSAIDS may have a profound effect on kidney function and glomerular filtration rate; some elderly people, especially those with cardiac or renal disease, are very sensitive to them and might develop a rapid rise in serum creatinine. This should be monitored very carefully. Strong NSAIDs might also have a profound effect on the hips, giving rise to the so-called indomethacin or NSAID hip. Probably because sensation is inhibited, hip joint disease can then become rapidly destructive.

Corticosteroids may induce or aggravate pathological changes, to which the elderly are highly susceptible. In polymyalgia, doses of 7.5 mg or even 5 mg prednisolone over a long period may induce diabetes mellitus and aggravate osteoporosis.

In a few patients D-penicillamine can induce myasthenia gravis, which stops if the drug is withdrawn. Here too the susceptibility has an immunogenetic basis, so that most patients are not at risk.

Conclusions

The factors briefly reviewed above are just the tip of an iceberg. Many others, as yet unknown, remain to be identified in the future. On the positive side, by contrast, the establishment of a rheumatic disease unit providing team support can trigger favourable responses – helping the patient to get back into society and to live as normally as possible, while minimising the risks of progressive joint damage and impairment of function. Knowledge of adverse trigger factors is vital if they are to be countered effectively.

References

BATCHELOR, J.R., WELSH, K.I., TINOURO et al (1980) Hydralazine-induced systemic lupus erythematosus influence of HLA-DR and sex on susceptibility. *Lancet i,* 1107–1109.

DEQUEKER, J. (1985) The relationship between osteoporosis and osteoarthritis. *Clin. Rheum. Dis. 11,* 271–296.

DEQUEKER, J., BURSSENS, A. and BOUILLON, R. (1982) Dynamics of growth hormone secretion in patients with osteoporosis and in patients with osteoarthrosis. *Horm. Res. 16,* 353–356.

DEQUEKER, J., DE PROFT, G. and FERIN, J. (1978b) The effect of long-term oestrogen treatment on the development of osteoarthrosis at the small hand joints. *Maturitas 1,* 27–30.

DEQUEKER, J., DECOCK, T., WALRAVENS, M. et al (1978a) A systemic survey of the HLA B27 prevalence in inflammatory rheumatic diseases. *J. Rheumatol. 5,* 452–459.

DEQUEKER, J., GORIS, P., UYTTERHOEVEN, R. (1983) Osteoporosis and osteoarthritis (osteoarthrosis): anthropometric distinctions. *JAMA 249,* 1448–1451.

DEQUEKER, J., VAN WANGHE, P. and VERDICKT, W. (1984) A systemic survey of HLA-A,B,C and D antigens and drug toxicity in rheumatoid arthritis. *J. Rheumatol. 11,* 282–286.

GEUSENS, P., DEQUEKER, J., VERSTRAETEN, A. et al (1986) Age-, sex-, and menopause-related changes of vertebral and peripheral bone: population study using dual and single photon absorptiometry and radiogrammetry. *J. Nucl. Med. 27,* 1540–1549.

KREMER, J.M., JUBIZ, W., MICHALEK, A. et al (1987) Fish-oil fatty acid supplementation in active rheumatoid arthritis. *Ann. Int. Med. 106,* 497–502.

VANDENBROUCKE, J.P., VALKENBORG, H., BOERSMA, A. et al (1982) Oral contraceptives and rheumatoid arthritis: further evidence for a preventive effect. *Lancet ii,* 831–842.

WOOLEY, P.H., GRIFFINS, J., PANAYS, G.S. et al (1980) HLA-DR antigens and toxic reactions to sodium aurothiomalate and D-penicillamine in patients with rheumatoid arthritis. *N. Engl. J. Med. 303,* 300–302.

Prognostically relevant clinical factors and strategies for therapeutic intervention

RAFFAELE NUMO

Community Medical Centre for Rheumatology, Bari, Italy

Summary

The three key issues in the management of the elderly rheumatic patient are the patient, the disease, and the drug. Together, they are influenced by the crucial role of ageing – which itself raises further questions. This paper seeks to identify factors of potential relevance for the prognosis and for the effects of therapeutic intervention in the elderly rheumatic patient.

Diagnosis and therapeutic management of the elderly rheumatic patient focuses attention on certain points – the disease itself, the drug to be used, and the background biological state of the patient. It also raises questions concerned with ageing: What causes it? What exactly does 'ageing' consist of? What is 'normal' ageing? How does it affect the onset of disease, its course, and the response to therapy? And are immunogenetics as relevant in rheumatic disorders of the elderly as in the young? In short, are there any factors which make it possible to predict the prognosis and/or the outcome of therapeutic intervention in the elderly rheumatic patient?

The current trend is to assume that the elderly patient is very likely to develop toxic side effects of therapy and to exhibit a poor clinical response. The latter assumption has been substantiated by extensive clinical data, which may be conveniently considered under three main headings – the patient, the disease, and drug treatment.

The patient

Every individual bears the 'scars' of any healing he has undergone in each of his biological systems, including the reticulo-endothelial system responsible for immune function.

There appears to be a higher incidence of certain rheumatic disorders among females than among males, notably rheumatoid arthritis (Fig. 1). The haplotype HLA A1 B8 (MAKINODAN and KAY, 1980) correlates with age only in the female. Moreover, B8 (which is known to be associated with autoimmune disturbances) in elderly females is responsible for reduced T-cell response (GREENBERG and YUNIS, 1978); this has not been found in the male.

Animal data, when extrapolated to humans, strongly suggest that major

29

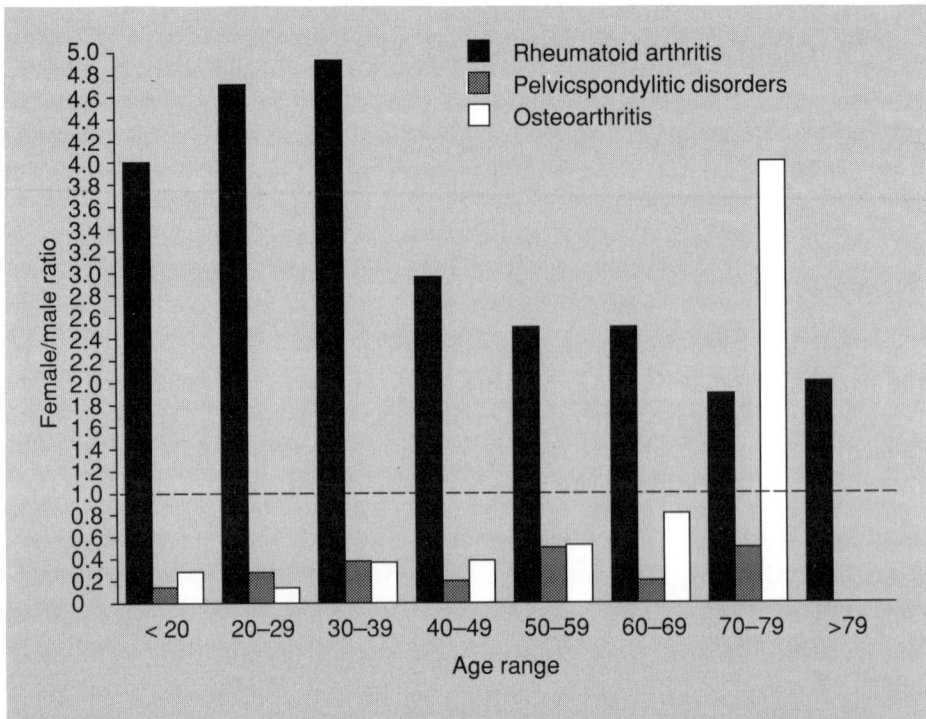

Fig. 1. Sex and age differences in the incidence of rheumatoid arthritis, seronegative spondyloarthropathies and osteoarthritis. Note that rheumatoid arthritis is consistently elevated well above the 1:1 ratio (dotted line), and only joined by osteoarthritis in women over 70. (Modified from AMOR, 1984).

histocompatibility complex (MHC) antigens can influence lifespan and immune reactivity by many different mechanisms. So far, no clear-cut haplotype has been implicated.

Thymus and thymic hormones do not appear to play a significant role in ageing, as the normal decay of their function does not run parallel to the lymphocyte population and function. There is great individual variability, depending partly on race and sex. As regards monoclonal antibodies, the relative proportion of pan T-cells (OK T3$^+$) and helper cells (OK T4$^+$) is normally reduced and that of the T-suppressor cells (OK T8$^+$) increased in elderly people. However, these findings are from peripheral blood, where redistribution cannot be investigated.

It has been demonstrated that stimulation of B-cells with T-dependent antigens decreases with age. The progressive and deviating antibodies produced with age are responsible for multidirectional polyclonal activation. This can give rise to some misleading clinical situations, where the presence of antigammaglobulin or of antinuclear factors can result in the underlying disease being misinterpreted.

Various phenomena have been described: different autoantibodies and circulating immune complexes (DELESPESSE et al, 1980); changes in the auto anti-idiotypic antibody response (GOIDL et al, 1986); reduction of mitogen response of peripheral-blood lymphocytes (HALLGREN et al, 1973). Moreover, delayed hypersensitivity is commonly impaired in the elderly (WALDORF et al, 1968). All these aspects combine to alert researchers and clinicians to the fact that immune tolerance and/or immune surveillance are slowing down.

Autoimmune disease. The autoantibodies produced with advancing age do not have any deleterious effect. For example, although the incidence of rheumatoid factor (RF) increases with age, the majority of elderly people positive for RF do not develop rheumatoid arthritis (RA).

Antilymphocyte antibodies occur more frequently in the elderly (LOKHORST et al, 1983); since immunity then decreases, they probably play a pathogenic role. MACKAY (1972) has stressed the possibility that life expectancy could be reduced in elderly people carrying autoantibodies. Moreover, HALLGREN and YUNIS (1977) have confirmed that a slowing down of suppressor cell function may reduce lifespan.

In older healthy subjects some plasma and cellular profiles are altered. High ESRs are not uncommon and are sometimes difficult to explain – slight increases in fibrinogen and haptoglobulin do not justify the change. IgM levels are normally reduced in the elderly.

Patients with elderly-onset rheumatoid arthritis (EORA) exhibit major differences with regard to the pattern of joint and systemic involvement and clinical aspects when compared with young-onset rheumatoid arthritis (YORA) patients (Fig. 2). Generally, the immunogenetic pattern in the elderly does not appear to be clear-cut and well differentiated; the increase in HLA DR4 is non-significant (38%, compared with 17% normally). TERKEL-TAUB and co-workers (1983) have described a significant increase in the frequency of CW3 among older RA patients and an eight-fold increase in the frequency of A25.

Sex hormones and genes. Sex hormones appear to play an important role in a variety of normal and pathological events, with the result that some disorders are more frequent in women and others in men:
1. Systemic lupus erythematosus (SLE) has a dramatically higher incidence in women than in men, the peak age for detection being after puberty. Late-onset-SLE, beginning around the time of the menopause, is milder. Disease severity appears to be influenced by factors which modify the normal estrogen balance, e.g. pregnancy and the contraceptive pill.
2. RA is more frequent in females than males during the reproductive years; the difference lessens with EORA.
3. Gout and Reiter's syndrome are more common in men than women.
4. Most of the seronegative spondyloarthropathies exhibit a preference for males, mainly in the younger age group (see Fig. 1).

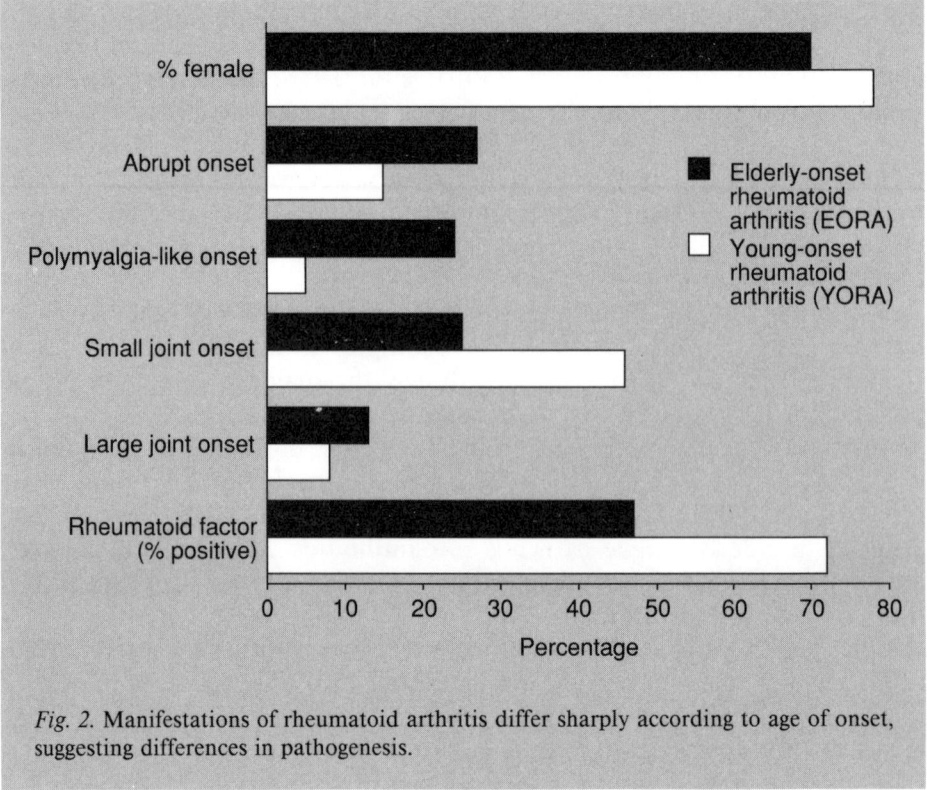

Fig. 2. Manifestations of rheumatoid arthritis differ sharply according to age of onset, suggesting differences in pathogenesis.

5. Polymyalgia rheumatica (PMR) is most frequently observed in menopausal females.

The contraceptive pill and pregnancy both provoke a flare-up of the clinical pattern in SLE, while RA patients experience some improvement with increased estrogen levels. The following points are of interest with regard to the influence of sex hormones on elderly-onset rheumatic diseases:

- Many sex steroids can exert an immunoregulatory effect which, if impaired, might be responsible for the appearance of diseases such as SLE and the flare-up of others, or might influence the course of chronic inflammatory conditions.
- Sex hormones exert their influence via the receptors widely present on the surface of many cell types in immune and non-immune populations.
- The antithesis between estrogens and androgens is highlighted when they are found to have an immunosuppressive effect via the selection of specific cellular subsets.
- A given disease may follow a different course under the same conditions in different patients. It is possible that the behavioural influence of sex steroids is related not to dose but to metabolites.

These data could account for the different patterns of the same rheumatic disease in both young and elderly patients. A given disease, such as RA, may

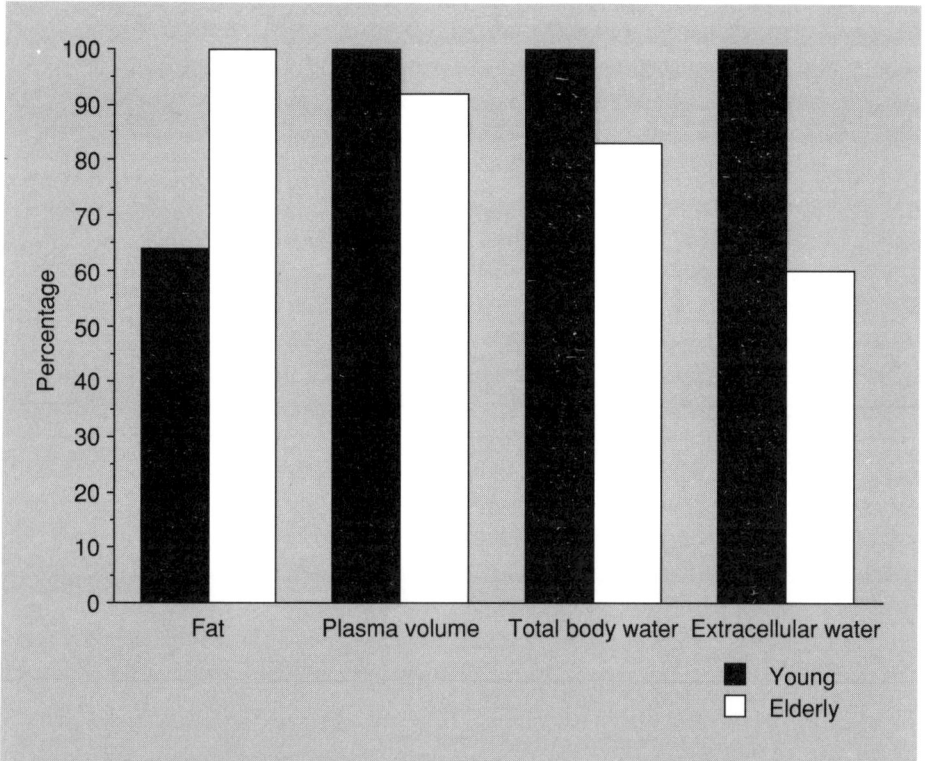

Fig. 3. Percentage changes in body fat and water with age. In the elderly, the rise in body fat and fall in body water mean that the distribution of most hydrophilic drugs is increased and that of lipophilic drugs decreased.

be unrecognisable because its onset, course and therapeutic response are so different from those normally associated with the condition.

Effect of ageing. Treatment of rheumatic diseases in the elderly may be hampered by the fact that various organs and systems are ageing and are therefore less flexible than they used to be. For example, the stomach of an elderly patient may not tolerate the full dosage of a non-steroidal anti-inflammatory drug (NSAID); gastrointestinal disturbances may thus develop. An undiagnosed atrophic gastritis can affect the rate of absorption of many molecules, limiting the effect of antirheumatic treatment. The kidney is characterised by reduced residual function, possibly developing into renal insufficiency. Ageing bone marrow is less tolerant to most antirheumatic drugs, the stem cell being particularly sensitive to drug toxicity. Finally, there is a higher ratio of fat to water in elderly people (Fig. 3), affecting drug distribution (NOVAK, 1972). Therefore distribution of most hydrophilic molecules is depressed, while that of lipophilic drugs is increased.

33

Even the most common rheumatic disorders are characterised by patterns in the elderly which differ from those in younger patients. Are they therefore the same diseases?

In general, the clinical onset of rheumatic disorders in the elderly is conditioned by many factors: ageing itself; likely concurrent diseases; possible concurrent medication (polypharmacy).

Due to the overlap of symptoms, it is sometimes difficult for the patient or doctor to distinguish a normal disturbance of ageing from a rheumatic sign or symptom. There is therefore a risk that some disorders will be underdiagnosed (e.g. polymyalgia) or even misdiagnosed (SLE can be mistaken for RA). There is also a tendency to concentrate on the rheumatic disorder and thus overlook concurrent pathological conditions.

Rheumatoid arthritis. Study of the literature has revealed that EORA has the following characteristics:
– a tendency to be localised in the shoulder joint (may be diagnosed as hand-shoulder syndrome or PMR)
– morning stiffness
– frequent polymyalgia rheumatica (PMR)-like onset
– frequently seronegative for rheumatoid factor but with sex and age differences (Fig. 4)
– ESR raised at onset
– few systemic manifestations, e.g. fever, weight loss
– onset frequently abrupt
– relatively more favourable prognosis and course
– more responsive than YORA to standard therapy with gold or disease-modifying antirheumatic drug (DMARD)
– very little erosion
– female:male ratio falling from 4:1 in favour of females
– proximal joint involvement
– less-deforming joint changes.

Some discrepancies exist between the different papers (TERKELTAUB et al, 1981, 1983 and 1984; DEAL et al, 1981 and 1985); these are attributable to the various populations investigated, but there are no striking racial differences in the onset or course of the disease.

ADLER et al (1982) in Israel reported that 13% of their rheumatoid patients had EORA; they found no patients in stage IV or class IV of the American Rheumatism Association classification, and a total absence of rheumatoid nodules. Their patients share the same features as our own population in southern Italy, where the rheumatoid factor (RF) differs in a normal population over 65, ranging from 8 to 20%. Although the frequency of RF is high, the incidence of rheumatoid nodules is very low. RF therefore does not appear to provoke the appearance of rheumatoid nodules or of other conditions such as vasculitis and neuropathy. According to findings from our

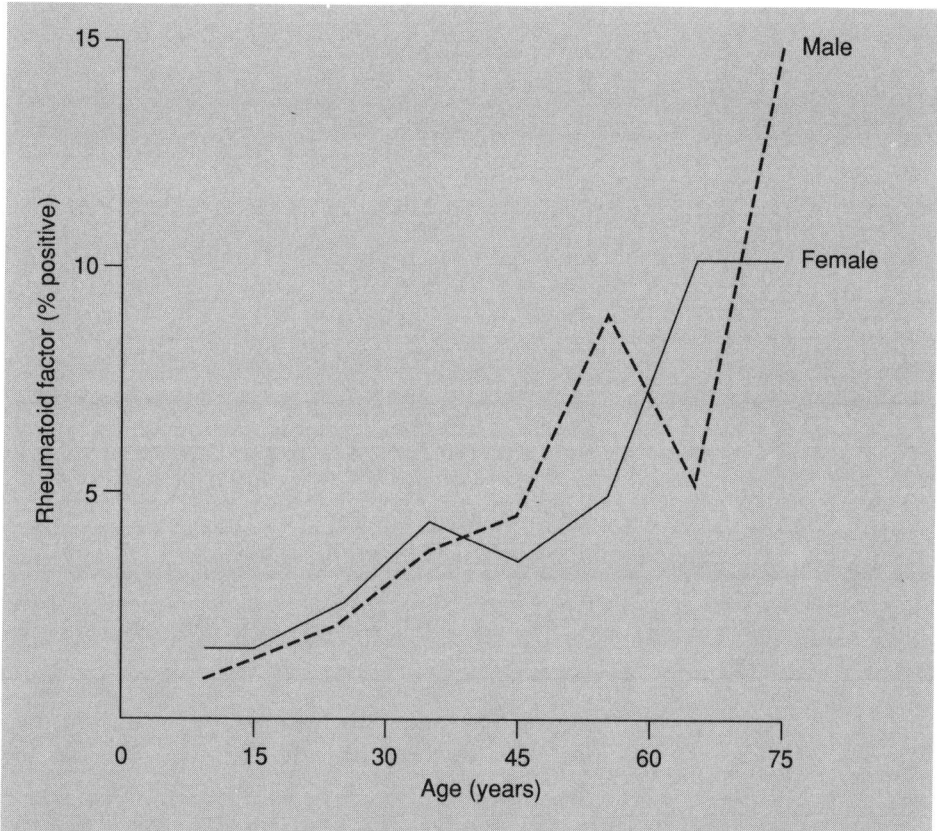

Fig. 4. Most cases of rheumatoid arthritis are negative for rheumatoid factor, but with major age and sex differences. Note the tendency for a positive response to rise from childhood throughout adult life and into old age, particularly in men.

population in southern Italy, RA tends to be seronegative and remain so for several years after its onset. But, in EORA, it frequently becomes seropositive as the disease progresses.

In a population investigated by Terkeltaub, 69% of EORA patients were seronegative for RF. Moreover, there was a high frequency of different RF plasma levels, in seemingly healthy subjects. The explanation for these apparently conflicting data could be that immunological reactivity was altered and there was a discrete change in plasma and clinical expression in older patients when challenged by a given stimulus.

'Seropositivity' seems to be a function of the duration of disease, both in young and old patients. There is certainly a distinction between seropositive and seronegative EORA. In the latter, the prognosis is good, there is less tendency to joint erosion, a good response to low doses of prednisolone and less risk of side effects to NSAIDs and DMARDs, all suggesting that a well-specified HLA haplotype exists which has not yet been clearly identified.

HEALEY (1986) has identified the following:
- Typical RA with or without nodules and RF
- Sjögren syndrome with RF, arthritis of the wrists and hands, and mild progression
- A PMR-like clinical picture with absence of RF and erosion but with marked morning stiffness.

Further immunogenetic data are needed to confirm these distinctions.

In EORA, there is often a discrepancy between a persistently elevated ESR and slightly altered inflammation indices, despite total absence of joint inflammation. Further investigations are needed to explain the possibility of superimposed or concurrent hidden infections, mainly in patients treated long term with steroids.

Recent data suggest that previous concurrent tuberculosis may exacerbate the course of RA, although no widely confirmed results are available as to the possible role of both previous and concurrent tuberculosis in EORA. Some constituents of the mycobacterium may indeed act as an adjuvant polyclonal factor, increasing autoantibody production in the elderly.

Connective tissue diseases. These appear to be underdiagnosed, particularly in the early stages.

The incidence of late-onset SLE is decreased in women and relatively increased in men (BALLOU et al, 1982), due to the influence of sex hormones. The clinical pattern is very similar in both sexes, when matched for age and duration of disease. It is characterised by a reduced incidence and severity of skin manifestations, alopecia and polyarthritis; by less severe involvement of the kidney (HOCHBERG et al, 1985); and, to a lesser degree, by a reduction of complement (WILSON et al, 1981). On the other hand, involvement of peripheral nerves and lung is more frequent and severe in older patients, while secondary Sjögren's syndrome also appears more often. In general, SLE is less severe in the elderly than in the younger population, and requires a low dose of steroid; in many cases satisfactory results can be obtained with chloroquine alone.

Dermatopolymyositis (DMPM) is associated in elderly females with a malignant condition; the typical skin lesions suggest a possible hidden neoplasm, but this has not yet been confirmed (CALLEN, 1984; FELDMAN et al, 1983).

Drug treatment

The use of both NSAIDs and DMARDs is a particular problem in elderly patients. Many factors influence the pharmacokinetics and pharmacodynamics of the drugs used – the modified tissue response, impaired clearance from the liver and kidney, and the altered rate of distribution between muscle and fat, among others. These factors do not preclude the use of these drugs, but underline the need for careful clinical monitoring of patients, so as to detect toxicity as early as possible. In general, the response of elderly rheumatic patients to NSAIDs is not significantly different from that of younger patients. Increased toxicity is the main problem, attributable to altered distribution, metabolism and excretion.

Which elderly patients are at high risk of developing side effects with NSAIDs? Those with concurrent metabolic disturbances experience a higher incidence of renal complications, though those with raised blood creatinine do not. Water retention occurs in the elderly – regardless of creatinaemia and urea nitrogen values – if there is an imbalance between sodium and potassium, suggesting local impairment of the prostaglandin/angiotensin II balance. Unconfirmed data (TAGGART and ALDERDICE, 1982) suggest that small debilitated women are at especially high risk of adverse hepatic and renal reactions to benoxaprofen.

The incidence of unwanted skin manifestations is highest among the overweight elderly, due to enterohepatic recirculation in mild liver dysfunction or to altered function of liver and bladder.

No correlation has been found between the severity of the clinical disease and the incidence of side effects, though HURWITZ (1969) reported an incidence of adverse reactions in elderly patients in their 70s seven times greater than in a matched group of patients in their 20s. Polymedication, particularly with strong cyclooxygenase inhibitors in association with antidiabetics and/or antihypertensives, increases the risk of side effects, as does diabetes itself.

Women appear to be more frequently affected than men by haematological side effects, while patients with coagulation defects are at a greater risk of haemorrhagia.

DMARDs appear to be less effective in the elderly, while exposing them to greater risks. The choice of which DMARD to prescribe is influenced by:
- life expectancy
- concurrent medication, and
- the possibility of poor compliance for social and mental reasons.

It is currently deemed justifiable to prescribe corticosteroids, since they are well tolerated, are effective at a lower dose than in younger people and have rather less serious side effects. On the other hand, the potential oncogenetic risk of some DMARDs when given long term is less in the elderly, whose life expectancy is reduced.

It has been thought that injectable gold salts are less active and more toxic in the elderly; however, this has been refuted by KEAN et al (1983), who found no significant difference between young and elderly patients as regards either efficacy or toxicity.

Conclusions

Disease-modifying drugs are acceptable in elderly people, provided contraindications are heeded. This becomes all the more important as mean lifespan increases.

Long-term, low-dose steroids may be used in the elderly, particularly if recurrent or superimposed infection is present.

Major concerns about the use of NSAIDs can be overcome by ensuring that the dose is as low as possible while still being therapeutically active. To date there are laboratory tests or clinical features which permit early detection of side effects on the liver and kidney. NSAIDs with a long half-life should not be used indiscriminately or self-prescribed because of the risk of accumulation.

References

ADLER, S.J., MORLEY, A.A. and SESHADRI, R.S. (1982) Reduced lymphocyte colony formation with age. *Clin. Exp. Immunol. 49*, 129.

AMOR, B. (1984) Consequences of arthritis in the elderly. In: *Nonsteroidal Antiinflammatory Agents in the Elderly*, p. 40. Eular, Basle.

BALLOU, S.P., KHAN, M.A. and KUSHENER, I. (1982) Clinical features of systemic lupus erythematosus. Differences related to race and age of onset. *Arthritis Rheum. 25*, 55–60.

CALLEN, J.P. (1984) Myositis and malignancy. *Clin. Rheum. Dis. 10*, 117–130.

DEAL, C.L., GOLDENBERG, D.L., MEENAN, R.F. et al (1981) Elderly onset rheumatoid arthritis: a comparison with earlier onset, matched for disease duration. *Arthritis Rheum. 24*, 599.

DEAL, C.L., MEENAN, R.F., GOLDENBERG, D.L. et al (1985) The clinical features of elderly-onset rheumatoid arthritis. *Arthritis Rheum. 28*, 987.

DELESPESSE, G., GAUSSET, P.H., SARFATI, M. et al (1980) Circulating immune complexes in old people and in diabetics: correlations with autoantibodies. *Clin. Exp. Immunol. 40*, 96.

FELDMAN, D., HOCHBERG, M.C., ZIZIC, T.M. et al (1983) Cutaneous vasculitis in adult polymyositis/dermatomyositis. *J. Rheumatol. 40*, 85.

GOIDL, E.A., GOOD, R.A., SISKIND, G.W. et al (1986) Studies of human responses in mice prone to autoimmune disorders. II. Decreased down-regulation by auto-anti-idiotype antibody in autoimmune-prone mice. *Cell. Immunol. 101*, 281–289.

GREENBERG, L.J. and YUNIS, E.J. (1978) Histocompatibility determinants, immune responsiveness and aging in man. *Fed. Proc. 37*, 1258–1262.

HALLGREN, H.M., BUCKLEY, C.E., GILBERTSEN, V.A. et al (1973) Lymphocyte phytohemagglutinin responsiveness, immunoglobulins and autoantibodies in ageing humans. *J. Immunol. 111*, 1101–1107.

HALLGREN, H.M. and YUNIS, E.J. (1977) Suppressor lymphocytes in young and aged humans. *J. Immunol. 118*, 2004–2008.

HEALEY, L.A. (1986) A clinical picture similar to polymyalgia rheumatica with no rheumatoid factor, marked morning stiffness. *Arthritis Rheum. 29*, 149.

HOCHBERG, M.C., BOYD, R.E., AHEARN, J.M. et al (1985) Systemic lupus erythematosus: a review of clinico-laboratory features and immunogenetic markers in 150 patients with emphasis on demographic subsets. *Medicine (Baltimore) 64*, 285–295.

HURWITZ, N. (1969) Predisposing factors in adverse reactions to drugs. *Br. Med. J. 1*, 536–539.

KEAN, W.F., BELLAMY, N. and BROOKS, P.M. (1983) Gold therapy in the elderly rheumatoid patient. *Arthritis Rheum. 6*, 705–711.

LOKHORST, H.M., VANDERLINDEN, J.A., SCHUZMAN, H.J. et al (1983) Immune function during aging in man: relation between serological abnormalities and cellular immune status. *Eur. J. Clin. Invest. 12*, 109.

MAKINODAN, T. and KAY, M.M.B. (1980) Age influence on the immune system. In: *Advances in Immunology*, Vol. 29, p. 287 (Ed. F. Dixon). Academic Press, New York.

NOVAK, L.P. (1972) Aging, total body potassium, fat free mass, red cell mass in males and females between the ages of 18 and 85 years. *J. Gerontol. 27*, 438.

TAGGART, H.M. and ALDERDICE, J.M. (1982) Fatal cholestatic jaundice in elderly patients taking benoxaprofen. *Br. Med. J. 284,* 1372.

TERKELTAUB, R., DECARY, F. and ESDAILE, J. (1984) An immunogenetic study of older age onset rheumatoid arthritis of the aged. *Br. Med. J. 11,* 147–149.

TERKELTAUB, R., ESDAILE, J., DECARY, F. et al (1981) Late onset rheumatoid arthritis. *Arthritis Rheum. 24,* 100.

TERKELTAUB, R., ESDAILE, J., DECARY, F. et al (1983) A clinical study of older age rheumatoid arthritis with comparison to a younger onset group. *J. Rheumatol. 10,* 418–424.

WALDORF, D.S., WILLKENS, R.F. and DECKER, J.L. (1968) Impaired delayed hypersensitivity in an aging population. Association with antinuclear reactivity and rheumatoid factor. *JAMA 203,* 831–834.

WILSON, H.L., HAMILTON, M.E., SPYKER, D.A. et al (1981) Age influences the clinical and serologic expressions of systemic lupus erythematosus. *Arthritis Rheum. 24,* 1230–1235.

Prescribing for the elderly rheumatic patient

GEORGE NUKI
Rheumatic Diseases Unit, University of Edinburgh,
Northern General Hospital, Edinburgh, UK

Summary

Many physiological and biochemical functions decline in the elderly, with falls in plasma albumin concentration, total body water and lean body mass, accompanied by a relative increase in total body fat. Age-related decreases in hepatic, renal and CNS functions and in immune responsiveness are also features of the normal ageing process, though variable in degree. While the age-related decline in hepatic function is not generally associated with clinically important effects, the decreases in renal bloodflow and glomerular filtration can reduce excretion significantly. Many elderly people have multiple pathology, need to take more drugs, and are therefore liable to more side effects. Their ability to recover from adverse reactions may also be impaired. Reporting of symptoms and treatment compliance tend to become unreliable.

All these factors influence the choice of analgesic, anti-inflammatory and disease-modifying drugs – and serve to emphasise the importance of avoiding high-risk agents in high-risk cases. The implications for prescribing extend to the education of primary care physicians and to the marketing policies of pharmaceutical companies.

Physicians in general are faced with an increasingly elderly population. It is estimated that by the year 2050 there will be 16 million Americans over the age of 85, with corresponding figures for Europe. In view of the multimorbidity and associated polypharmacy often encountered in the elderly, it is important to consider the strategies for therapeutic intervention.

Ageing is associated with a linear decrease in a variety of physiological and biochemical functions, which must not themselves be mistaken for disease (ROWE, 1984). Age-related decreases in cardiac output, vital capacity, immune responsiveness and CNS functioning, as well as renal and hepatic function, are all features of the normal ageing process (Fig. 1), although the individual variability of these age-related changes is one of their most important characteristics.

Physiological and metabolic changes

Normality, in the sense of generality, does not however imply that age-related physiological changes are totally harmless and free from clinical significance.

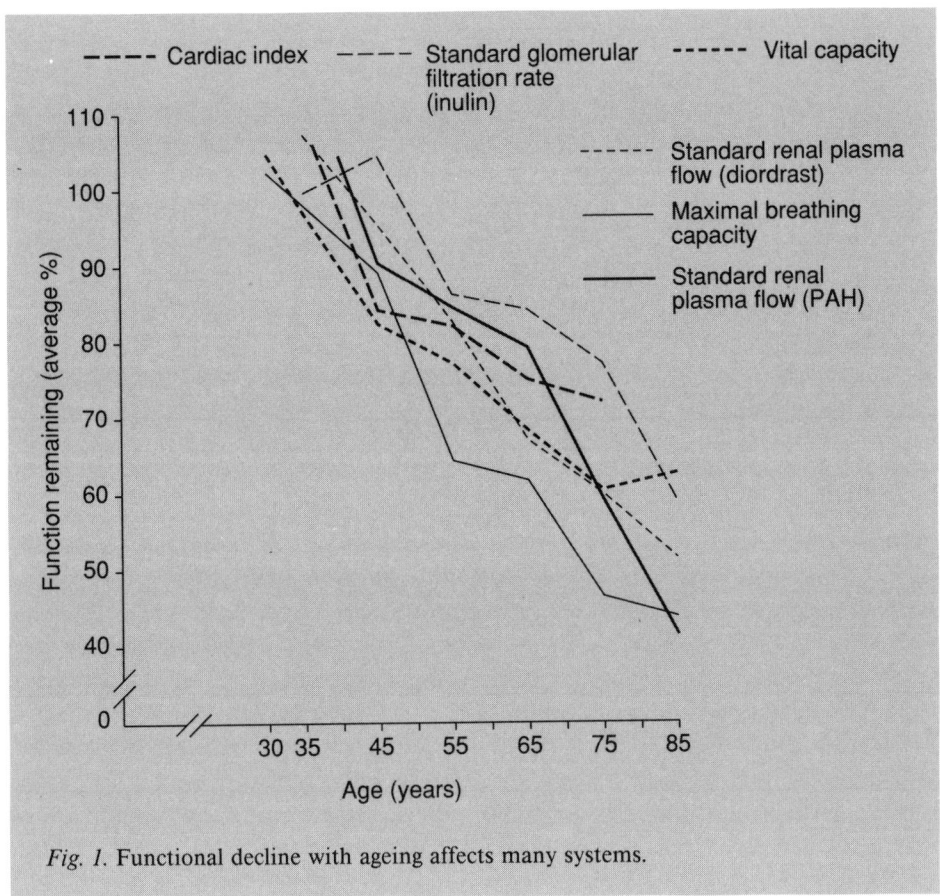

Fig. 1. Functional decline with ageing affects many systems.

In particular, the pharmacokinetics of drugs can be profoundly affected by age-related physiological changes. Absorption is generally not affected, but decreases in total body water and lean body mass associated with an increase in body fat result in an increase in the volume of distribution of hydrophilic agents such as paracetamol (Fig. 2).

Age-related decreases in plasma albumin can result in transient increases in free drug concentrations of non-steroidal anti-inflammatory drugs (NSAIDs) which are normally highly protein bound, especially in elderly patients receiving multiple drugs, but this is not usually a problem during chronic dosing. Ageing is associated with a decline in phase I oxidative hepatic metabolism, with decreased oxidation, reduction, hydrolysis and demethylation. Conjugation and glucuronidation in phase II are also reduced (Fig. 3). However, the functional reserve of the liver is considerable, and clinically important age-related effects on the first-pass metabolism of antirheumatic drugs do not occur.

By contrast, age-related declines in renal bloodflow, glomerular filtration and tubular function do have very important implications for the use of prosta-

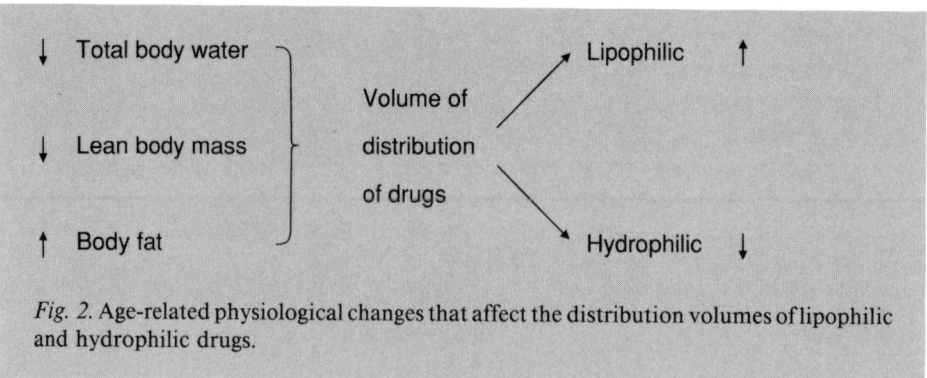

Fig. 2. Age-related physiological changes that affect the distribution volumes of lipophilic and hydrophilic drugs.

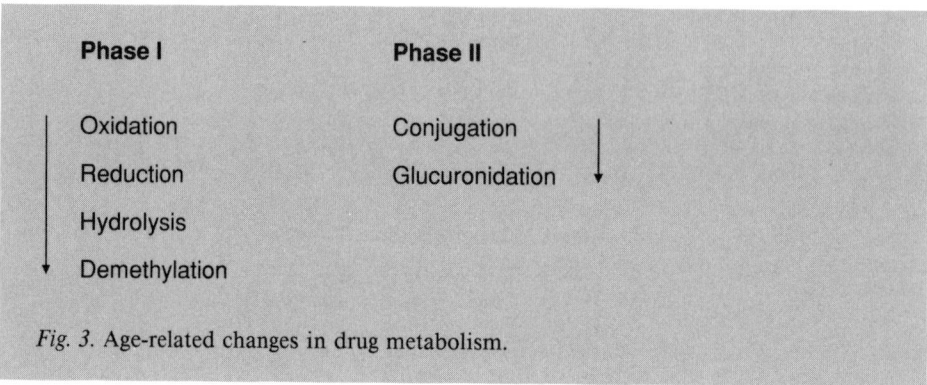

Fig. 3. Age-related changes in drug metabolism.

glandin synthetase inhibitors, disease-modifying antirheumatic drugs and allopurinol. On average, renal function is halved by the age of 90, even in the absence of renal disease.

Many of the anti-inflammatory drugs widely used at present have an unchanged elimination half-life in the elderly. These include diclofenac, fenbufen, flurbiprofen, indomethacin and piroxicam. (With azapropazone, benoxaprofen, diflunisal and paracetamol the elimination half-life is increased.) Theoretically at least, there is no reason to reduce dosage of these drugs in elderly people with renal insufficiency or a decline in renal function.

Illness clustering and adverse drug reactions

At least as important as age-related physiological changes is the clustering of illness in the elderly. Multiple pathology is the rule rather than the exception. A community survey in the 1960s of people over the age of 65 revealed an average of 3.5 important disabling conditions per person of which neither they nor the doctor were in many cases aware (WILLIAMSON et al, 1964).

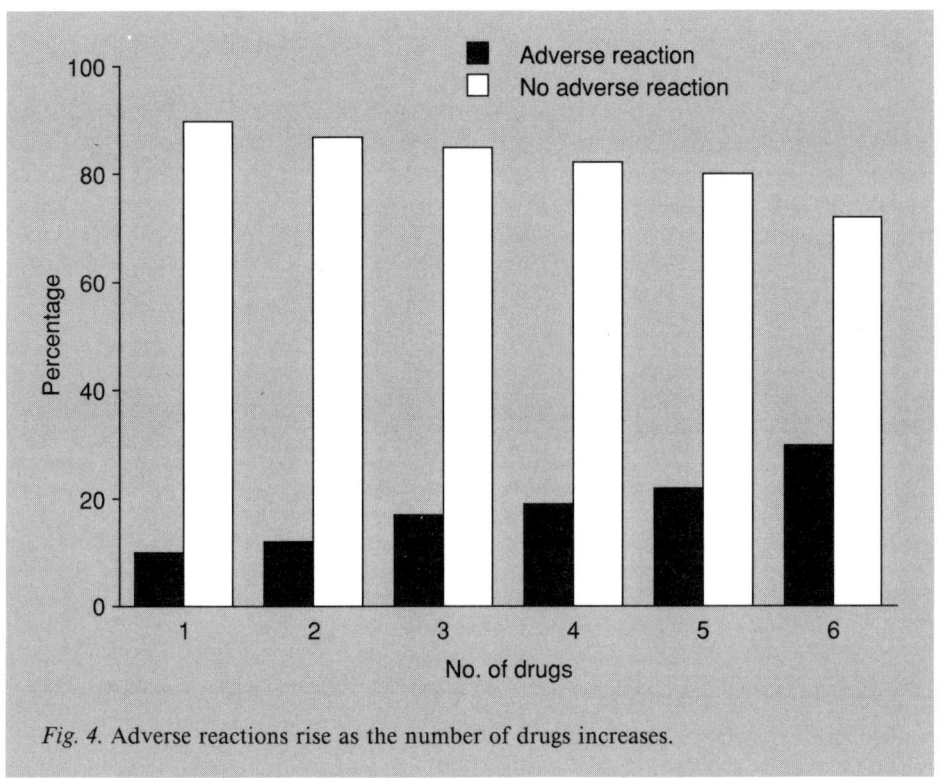

Fig. 4. Adverse reactions rise as the number of drugs increases.

Polymorbidity leads to polypharmacy and an increase in the prevalence of adverse drug events in the elderly (Fig. 4). Important examples in patients with rheumatic diseases include NSAID-induced acute cardiac or renal failure in elderly patients with preceding cardiac or renal insufficiency, diuretic-induced gout in patients with preceding hyperuricaemia, and symptomatic osteoporotic collapse in steroid-treated patients with longstanding renal or hepatic disease. Stevens-Johnson syndrome may occur, but is unpredictable. Asthma and anaphylaxis are rare, but if they develop with one NSAID they will probably occur with others too. The doctor must also look out for drug interactions, and bear in mind the possibility of liver failure. Retrospective case-controlled studies of patients admitted to hospital with haematemesis and melaena due to gastric and duodenal ulcer suggest that the relative risk from NSAIDs is increased two- to four-fold in women over the age of 60, with an attributable risk of 22% (WALT et al, 1986).

Preliminary results from record linkage studies in Scotland suggest that one can identify high-risk drugs (Table I) as well as high-risk patients for gastro-intestinal haemorrhage; evidence is beginning to emerge that morbidity and mortality may be reduced by avoiding NSAIDs in elderly patients (Table II) with high-risk disease (Table III). When dealing with elderly people, it is desirable to look for alternative strategies to drug therapy. Clearly this has

Table I. Gastrointestinal events – differing rates linked to NSAID therapy among almost 26,000 patients. (From: Tayside Record Linkage Study, 1983).

NSAID	GI events	Relative risk	95% confidence
Osmosin (n=1161)	156	1.85	1.56–2.21
Indomethacin (n=5155)	608	1.60	1.45–1.76
Naproxen (n=8184)	859	1.40	1.29–1.52
Piroxicam (n=4427)	573	1.78	1.61–1.96
Ibuprofen (n=7032)	726	1.37	1.22–1.50

Table II. Risk of gastrointestinal events on NSAID therapy rises with age. (Over 26,000 patients from Tayside Record Linkage Study, 1983.) See Table I.

Age	<49	50–69	70–99
Patients	7926	10,395	7998
NSAID	278	765	963
Relative risk (95% confidence)	1.60 1.37–1.87	1.35 1.22–1.49	1.66 1.52–1.81
Attributable rate (95% confidence)	20/1000 ± 6	23/1000 ± 8	65/1000 ± 11

Table III. High-risk conditions in the elderly, requiring care in prescribing.

- Heart disease and incipient cardiac failure
- A history of dyspepsia, peptic ulceration or gastrointestinal bleeding
- Renal insufficiency or volume depletion
- Alcoholism, cirrhosis or serious impairment of liver function
- Low weight, general debility, senile or presenile dementia, and cerebrovascular disease

important implications for the modification of drug prescribing, the education of primary care physicians and the marketing policies of pharmaceutical companies.

Cascades of iatrogenic disease are particularly likely to occur when the underlying multiple pathology goes unrecognised. NSAID → oedema → digoxin + diuretic → hypokalaemia → added potassium → anorexia + GI upset → hospitalisation is one such vicious spiral that is all too often seen in geriatric practice (BRAVERMAN, 1982). Impairment of homoeostasis is a characteristic of ageing, and an individual's ability to recover from adverse drug reactions such as NSAID-induced gastrointestinal haemorrhage, heart failure or acute renal insufficiency is significantly impaired, particularly when there is preceding gastrointestinal, cardiac or renal disease.

Clearcut examples of altered pharmacodynamics of antirheumatic drugs have not been so well documented, but there is some evidence that elderly bone marrow is more susceptible to drugs that can occasionally induce aplastic anaemia and that elderly patients with renal insufficiency are particularly dependent on renal prostaglandin for maintaining renal bloodflow and particularly susceptible to prostaglandin synthetase inhibitors with potent effects on renal prostanoids.

Multimorbidity can lead to disease-disease interactions as well as adverse interactions with drugs. Urinary tract infection, for example, not infrequently leads to incontinence in elderly arthritics whose mobility is impaired. Illness behaviour also tends to differ in the elderly, with widespread under-reporting of symptoms and unreliable treatment compliance.

Strategies for therapeutic intervention in elderly patients with rheumatic diseases demand careful consideration of risks and benefit in relation to the overall quality of life.

Guidelines for prescribing

Important general principles that should be considered before prescribing any drug to the elderly include:
  1. *Sensible assessment of the cause of the problem to be treated.*
  2. *Thorough diagnostic appraisal of multiple pathology and its implications for drug therapy.*
  3. *Accurate and complete information about the patient's drug history.*
  4. *Sound knowledge of the pharmacology of the drugs prescribed and their possible interactions.*
  5. *Problem-oriented approach to therapy.*
  6. *Careful titration of drug dosage to patient response.*
  7. *Use of smaller doses of drugs in the elderly.*
  8. *Rigorous and repeated simplification of therapeutic regimens.*
  9. *Keen and constant awareness of the possibility of iatrogenic disease.*
  10. *Discontinuation of unnecessary medication.*
  11. *Avoidance of drugs in high-risk patients.*

12. *Care in choosing the safest drugs first where possible and avoiding high-risk agents.*

13. *Sanguine appraisal of prospects for compliance and consequences of non-compliance.*

In choosing an NSAID for an elderly person, safety and convenience should be major considerations, and it is essential to have a measure of the patient's renal function. Elderly females appear to carry a greater risk of serious adverse reactions than males (30%, compared with 25%), though the high-risk conditions listed in Table III apply to both sexes.

Care should be taken to try and avoid agents with a high incidence of side effects involving the central nervous system (high-dosage aspirin and indomethacin), drugs that are particularly prone to cause fluid retention (high-dosage aspirin, phenylbutazone, azapropazone and indomethacin) and highly gastrotoxic drugs. Since gastrointestinal bleeding and perforation are the major serious adverse reactions caused by NSAIDs, large-scale record-linkage studies are now required to assess the relative risk of individual agents. Clinically important drug interactions with NSAIDs include those with oral anticoagulants, sulphanylurea hypoglycaemic agents, diclofenac, lithium, methotrexate and salicylates, uricosuric agents and all classes of hypotensive drugs. Interactions between salicylates and probenacid and sulphinpyrazone are also well known.

Low-dosage systemic corticosteroids are sometimes indicated when a patient's physical independence is being threatened by active inflammatory disease, but local intra-articular and soft-tissue injections are important practical alternative strategies that should always be considered.

Second-line, disease-modifying and immunosuppressive drugs can occasionally be useful in selected elderly patients with severe inflammatory joint disease, but modification of the patient's environment and the possibility of supportive treatment other than drugs always need to be borne in mind. Voltaire had a point when he commented that 'Doctors pour drugs of which they know little, to cure diseases of which they know less, into human beings of whom they know nothing.' We need to consider the elderly patient as a whole, and treat him or her accordingly.

References

BRAVERMAN, A. M. (1982) Therapeutic considerations in prescribing for elderly patients. *Eur. J. Rheumatol. Inflam. 5*, 289–293.

NUKI, G. and BURLEY, L. (1984) Nonsteroidal analgesic anti-inflammatory drugs in the elderly. In: *The Ageing Process: Therapeutic Implications*, pp. 207–225 (Eds. R.N. Butler and A.G. Bearn). Raven Press, New York.

ROWE, J.W. (1984) Physiologic changes with age and their clinical relevance. In: *The Ageing Process: Therapeutic Implications*, pp. 41–50 (Eds. R.N. Butler and A.G. Bearn). Raven Press, New York.

WALT, R., KATSCHINSKI, B., LOGAN, R. et al (1986) Rising frequency of ulcer perforation in elderly people in the United Kingdom. *Lancet i*, 489–492.

WILLIAMSON, J., STOKOE, I.H., GRAY, S. et al (1964) Old people at home – their unreported needs. *Lancet i*, 1117–1120.

Perspective
Caring for the elderly rheumatic patient

GEORGE E. EHRLICH

Medical Department, Ciba-Geigy Ltd, Basle, Switzerland

Care of the elderly must always take account of their physical, physiological, and psychological characteristics. Administration of medications presents special problems. In addition to differences in metabolism of drugs, age-related changes in memory often make it difficult for patients to remember the dosage to be taken, with all the consequences of under- or over-dosage. The patient's age also contributes to surgical decisions, as anaesthesia is less well tolerated and recovery from anaesthesia and surgery tends to be slower. Musculoskeletal impairment may inhibit salutary responses to physical therapy. Transport is often a particular problem for elderly individuals, limiting not only social activities but also the availability of medical care, and probably represents the major reason for social and medical isolation. Reduced budgets commonly compound these problems. For all their advantages, retirement communities and homes for the aged may isolate elderly individuals from the wider community in some countries; in others, family, community, and social customs continue to integrate the individual but result in other problems and burdens.

It may be appropriate here to cite Cephalus, who answers Socrates: *When they meet, most of the members of our group lament, longing for the pleasures of youth and reminiscing about sex, about drinking bouts and feasts and all that goes with things of that sort. They take it as hard as though they were deprived of something very important and have been living well but now are not even alive. Some also bewail the abuse that old age receives from relatives, and in this key they sing a refrain about all the evils old age has caused them. But these men do not put a finger on the cause. For if this were the cause, I too would have suffered these same things in so far as they depend on old age – and so would everyone else who has come to this point in life. But of these things and of those that concern relatives, there is one certain cause, not old age, but the character of human beings. If they are balanced and good tempered, even old age is only moderately troublesome. And if they are not, then both age and youth alike are likely to be hard...*

Yet, today, whatever their character, elderly people are potential victims of street crime – particularly as they cannot fight back and cannot run away. It is also true that social factors and habits acquired through a lifetime in part dictate how we spend our later years. While various studies have demonstrated that many people who live to a ripe old age enjoy surprisingly good health, we now recognise osteoarthritis as a consequence of life-long subclinical development. Care of the elderly needs to be considered in this perspective. Only in recent years has the specialty of paediatrics been recognising the developmental aspects of childhood that influence adult life. Now we are beginning to perceive earlier in adult life the factors that predispose to later disability. It has, for example, been reported elsewhere at this congress that rural inhabitants of an area in southern Africa, where parasite infestation and high immunoglobulin levels are present, have very low rates of rheumatoid arthritis (about 0.002%). But when these people migrate to the cities, the rheumatoid arthritis rate rises sharply (to about 2%). Some factors other than genetics must be playing a part in this thousand-fold rise.

Some of the factors predisposing to such differences may be relatively minor in themselves. Osteoarthritis of the hip, for instance, is relatively uncommon in countries where people normally sit cross-legged, being almost never seen among Mexican Indians. It is also less common in people who traditionally squat than in countries where almost everybody sits on chairs. Such observations suggest cause and effect, but suggestion is not enough. In caring for the elderly rheumatic patient we have to know what treatment is most appropriate and how it may be safely given. Equally we must learn more about the earlier causes of rheumatic disorders and diseases in the elderly, with a view to developing timely preventive measures in the future.